OWN YOUR HEALTH

CHANGE YOUR DESTINY

Ancient knowledge made
simple

Rita Panahi, L.Ac., Dipl.O.M.

Copyright 2017 by Rita Panahi

ISBN: 978-0-9996648-0-3

First Edition: Nov 2017

10% of all author royalties are donated to the poor

"Your Health is the greatest Treasure.

You must make taking care of it a Priority"

– Rita Panahi, L.Ac.

To the Reader

The content in this book should not be followed without first consulting a health care professional. If you have any medical conditions requiring attention, you should consult with your health care professional regularly, regarding possible modifications of the steps in this book. If you have allergies to certain foods, avoid them.

Dedicated to:

My family

Table of Contents

Introduction

With new diets coming out every month, it's sometimes hard to know what to follow. Instead of giving you a diet to follow, which can sometimes get complicated, I want to give you the most important basic guidelines to take a step toward health for the long run.

I will not be using complicated terminology to scare you, but instead, I will provide an explanation using down-to-earth terms that are simple and make sense, helping you to understand the basic fundamentals of how to be healthy.

I have a Masters in Chinese Medicine, a 5000-year-old medicine, which in ancient times was used as a form of preventative medicine, meaning that if you did the right things before you got sick, the chances of getting sick would be greatly reduced. Yet in our world today, many come to learn about Chinese Medicine only after they have tried everything under the sun and exhausted all their options with nothing having worked, and are surprised to find the benefits of Chinese Medicine and healing naturally. My motto is "Food is Your First Medicine". I teach my patients to not be dependent on medications, herbs, or supplements if they can help it. We are eating every day. What we eat and drink is what makes up our body and gives it the proper fuel. However, we were never taught how to eat right when we were young and are surprised when we fall ill when we are older, or sometimes even when we are young.

I turned my own life around following these steps and I share them with all of my patients to keep them healthy and on the right track. It's not always easy to change 20 years, 30 years or 50 years of life habits around, but it's never too late and it doesn't all need to change overnight. It simply needs to begin with one step. Just do one thing, whatever is easiest for you in this book, for a few weeks. After you have changed one thing, then add another new habit for a few weeks. This is the best way to make changes and have them be long lasting so that it does not backfire on you. Be easy on yourself and take it one step at a time. Know that even one step will help you towards a healthier you. And sometimes just one step can completely turn your life and health around. I have seen it so often, that when a person has changed only one thing, for example drinking the right amount of water or drinking only room temperature water, almost all of their symptoms changed within a couple of weeks! So even though the things I share are simple, they are so important that they can turn your life and health around. In search of the new, often we forget the basic simplicities of life. Try the changes and give it a try for 3 months. Of course, the more of the steps you follow, the greater your results in the long run but even just one step is well worth the change. Don't be fooled by the simplicity of the steps either. They can have a powerful impact on your health, as I have seen over and over again, in my own life and in those of my patients. Many who have followed these steps, not only have found their health condition and energy improve, but they have had the added bonus of naturally losing weight. The more empowered you are to take your health into your own hands, and understand the power of foods and drinks and the choices you make, the less you will need to see a doctor. Remember, Your Body is Your Treasure. Make it a priority. Take good care of it. Your health is what will create your quality of life in the long run.

"In search of a million dollars, we forget the million dollars that we already have, our Health.

There is nothing more valuable and more worth our time than that."

- Rita Panahi, L.Ac.

I Want to be Healthy!

Let us begin to take care of the million dollars that we have – our body, our health, our true wealth

#1

The Temperature of What You Drink

Drink water (and all drinks) at room temperature or warm – NOT cold.

No matter how hot or cold it is outside, the inside of your body has to maintain a certain temperature to function optimally. When you drink cold or iced drinks or water, the same way that your body contracts when jumping into a cold pool is how your insides respond to the cold entering your mouth and moving down into your stomach. Cold contracts all the organs it passes through and slows down your digestion and metabolism. Your body needs to use up its energy to bring the stomach back to the proper temperature to be able to function well again.

Your stomach releases the enzymes when it is at its optimum temperature. In all that time, food that is inside the stomach needs to sit until it can be digested.

In Chinese Medicine, warming up the body requires energy, or qi. The body does not have an infinite amount of energy, so using this energy to bring the body back to its ideal temperature inside, and on a regular basis daily, is a waste of energy and weakens the body in the long run.

Drinking cold water and drinks is often a cause of many digestive issues and even weight gain. If you find that water is difficult to drink at room temperature because of its lack of taste, add a little lemon to it or just a small amount of an organic juice to give it a bit of flavor.

#2

Amount of Water

Drink plenty of clean, pure water throughout the day (about 50% of your body weight in ounces). Your body needs water for all of its functions, to bring nutrients into the cells and to clear out toxins. Your blood is approximately 70% water. It is the H-hydrogen and O-oxygen molecules of water, H2O, that support the waste removal and nutrient absorption out of and into the cells in the metabolic process. The importance of water is extremely underestimated. If you weigh 130 lbs, you need to drink at least 65 oz of pure water daily. It is best if the water is still water (not carbonated), because carbonated water does not hydrate you the same. Do not count juices and coffee or even some teas towards your water intake. Juices are often filled with concentrated sugar, while coffee and some teas are more of a diuretic and pull more water out of your system. As such, only water is water.

A good way to remember how much you have had in a day is to fill a 64oz glass bottle every morning and take it to work or leave it on the kitchen counter if you are home. By the end of the day, you can see how much you have actually drunk. It is hard to keep track objectively everyday as you get busy with errands, work and family.

If you do a lot of physical activity either through your work or exercise, then the amount of water that you drink needs to be even more, because you will be losing more water through sweating.

On a side note:

*Be sure to drink water out of glass bottles. Too often plastic bottles are left in the car, exposed to the heat of the sun. Plastic leaches chemicals into the water, mimicking the hormones of our body and throwing the body's hormonal system off balance.

*Be sure the quality of your water is good. Usually refrigerator filters are very weak, especially if the water source to the filter is not a very good one. Do research on the water quality in your area and if necessary buy a good quality water filter for your home.

#3

The Best Time to Drink Water

It is a good habit to drink water the moment you wake up, before breakfast, before tea, and before any snacks. Let water be your very first drink. It will begin your day with hydrating your body as well as helping to cleanse out any toxins.

When you are drinking water along with your food, it is best to drink it in smaller sips rather than a large gulp. Too much water with food dilutes the enzymes needed to do their job of breaking down the food and slows down your digestive process.

If you are trying to lose weight, drink water before you begin eating your meals. Doing so will help you to eat smaller portions. Sometimes a signal for thirst is misunderstood as a signal for hunger. If you drink enough water throughout the day, you may find that you are not as hungry as you thought you were.

#4

Processed Foods Transformed

Avoid processed foods such as: sugar (it doesn't matter if it's white or brown), fast food, soda, milk-shakes, jello, candy, ice-cream, dessert, chips, pastries, energy drinks, chocolate, cakes, and donuts.

Most of these processed foods are filled with a large amount of sugar, food colorings and chemicals, and in truth offer very little nutritional value. There are so many healthier versions of what I call 'fun foods', 'comfort foods', 'energy-boosting foods'. My motto is, if you can't pronounce the name that's written in the list of the ingredients, it probably shouldn't be going into your body. If processed food requires so many additives to preserve it, it's not a food source that's filled with a life-force. Always read labels and look at the ingredients carefully. If you search online, you can find healthier versions of almost anything. Here are a few of my favorite simple recipes to try:

Craving Chips?

Healthy Chips – Cut up organic kale leaves, sweet potato or beets. Bake them in the oven with a little oil and salt (sometimes a hint of lemon) and make your own chips! You can add organic pumpkin seeds too. The oven temperature and cooking time varies for each. There are many recipes to choose from online.

Craving Ice Cream?

Healthy ice cream – Peel a very ripe organic banana and freeze it. Use it as your vanilla base. When you are craving ice cream, put the banana in a food processor (or Vitamix), add a little bit of organic almond milk, add in the flavoring of your choice, for example, organic dried blue berries, mangoes, pistachio, cacao nibs, or coconut, and mix it. And there you have your creamy ice cream!

Craving Chocolate?

Healthy Chocolate – use organic pitted dates, organic almonds and organic cacao powder. Take about 15 dates, 20-25 almonds, 1 tablespoon of cacao power. Mix all of the ingredients in a food processer. Let it mix until it becomes one mass that rotates in the food processor. When it's all well blended, scoop out small amounts, just enough to make small balls or cubes. Make the shape, sprinkle some organic shredded coconut flakes or more cacao powder on them and put them in a freezer. You can add other ingredients, such as other variations of nuts, or cinnamon.

#5

The Magic of Vegetables

Eat one large bowl of mixed steamed vegetables with one meal once a day! Many of you, when you hear the word vegetable think of salads. While lettuce does grow in the earth alongside zucchini, asparagus, carrots and all the rest of the veggies, it consists mainly of water and roughage for your body.

What I am referring to are all the rest of the vegetables, such as carrots, asparagus, broccoli, green string beans, cauliflower, brussel sprouts, yams, sweet potato, beets, arugula, kale, spinach, chard, bok choy, and cabbage, to name a few.

It always surprises me when I ask which vegetables someone eats, how few they mention, and sometimes, sadly enough, it can be none, when there are such a beautiful array of vegetables to choose from. We need to make friends with vegetables, encourage our family members to make friends with them, and accept that they are a very important part of the diet that is not given enough importance.

Remember that some of these vegetables are very hard to digest if they are eaten raw, especially for people with an already weakened digestive system. Those vegetables include for example kale, cabbage and broccoli. I find it best to lightly steam vegetables before eating. Every day have a large bowl of 2-3 different mixed vegetables, steamed.

If they are too bland for you, add a little olive oil at the end and a little Himalayan salt (if you don't have any contraindications to salt). Do this every day. Vegetables are filled with nutrients and in my opinion, apart from nourishing your body, they are like a broom that also clean out your intestines. No matter how frequently or infrequently you have a bowel movement, vegetables will help remove the debris that may be stuck to the intestinal walls without you knowing it.

"It's never too late to take steps

Towards making better, healthier choices"

- Rita Panahi, L.Ac

#6

Fake Energy. Real Energy.

Reduce your coffee intake. Coffee is a form of "fake" energy, causing your body to become even more depleted in the long run. If you are feeling tired, it's because your body is telling you it's tired and needs to rest. If you are wanting to keep going and not listen to your body, it's your choice, but in the long run you are depleting your body's resources by drinking coffee. When you eat something, it gives you real energy because of its nutrients (if it's a nutritious food). But coffee is a stimulant, which means that if you have only $10 in your account, it's making you think that you have $100. So you are spending $100 and going into the negative by $90. You may not notice it daily, but in the long run, it most definitely catches up with you, leading to many other types of ailments because the resources of your body have been depleted over time. When your body needs its resources to fight disease, it will have less resources to do so.

Rather than drinking coffee, or any stimulant for that matter, for energy, eat better instead, which strengthens your body at the root, providing you with true energy. Or why not try making a smoothie with fruits and vegetables that are rich with vitamins!

You could try for example: 1 banana, 1 pitted date, a handful of spinach or chard, ½ apple, organic food-based protein powder, and water. You can play around with this to make it to your liking, as long as you don't fill it with ice nor all fruits, but add some vegetables in there too to balance out the concentrated sugar. And be sure to drink it slowly! You wouldn't eat all of those vegetables in 1 minute, so drink it as if you were eating it.

#7

Chewing and Digestion

The digestive process begins in your mouth. Chew your food very well until it's liquid before swallowing. Chewing is the start of the digestive process. The enzymes in your mouth need to mix in with the food to start digestion. When you chew well, it makes it easier on your stomach to more fully digest your food as well. If you eat too fast, your body will not be able to break down your food effectively nor absorb the nutrients efficiently, in addition it leads to bloating and gas. Chewing well also slows you down so that you do not overeat.

#8

The Best Way to Eat Nuts

Nuts are a healthy food, but harder to digest. When eating nuts, it is best to soak them first for several hours, throw out that water, and then eat them. When you soak them first, it makes them easier to digest and be absorbed.

If you are trying to lose weight, eating too many nuts or nut butters on a daily basis can slow down this process, especially if your digestive system is already weak. And if you have had your gall bladder removed, it would be best to reduce your nut intake, as nuts are high in fat and bile from the gall bladder is what supports the digestion of fat.

On a side note: I have seen many problems in people's health steming from eating peanuts and peanut butter, such as itching, body rashes, congestion in the sinuses, constipation, headaches, menstrual pain, and heavy bleeding. If you are in the habit of eating peanuts, peanut butter, or peanut butter and jelly sandwiches, try to go without it for a few months and see how you feel.

#9

The Best Way to Eat Beans

Soak your beans overnight, drain the water, and rinse them before cooking. This not only reduces the cooking time, but also helps the beans become more easily digestible. Soaking beans helps to reduce gas, heartburn, reflux and bloating that is often an issue when eating them and a reason why many people avoid beans, though they are a great source of protein. As a general rule, larger beans are harder to digest and more prone to causing gas. If you are using canned beans, most likely they have not been soaked prior to being cooked and canned. It's best to buy dried organic beans and follow these steps before cooking.

#10

I Love Vegetable Juices

Juicing is a great way to get nutrients and cleanse the body. Cleansing should be a part of our routine on a regular basis throughout the year. We take showers on a daily basis, but we don't think that our body requires cleaning on the inside as well. Think of your car. If you do not take it for an oil change, change the brakes, change the fluids, or fill it with gas, after 20 years, 30 years, or more, what would happen? We rarely think of our body in the same way, imagining that it's invincible and we can put whatever we want in it, and it will just keep going.

It's very important to cleanse the body and vegetable juices are one of the best ways to do that. Start your morning 2-3x a week by drinking organic vegetable juice. You could mix carrots, beets, kale, chard, celery, parsley. Be creative. Remember, because it's a very high concentration of vegetables, always dilute it with some water and drink it slowly. You wouldn't be eating those vegetables in 1 minute, so drink it as if you were chewing it, slowly.

Vegetable juices are also wonderful for giving you energy, a much better choice than coffee.

On a side note: Avoid canned vegetable juices. They have added preservatives that will defeat the purpose of helping to cleanse your body of toxins.

Refrigerated organic vegetable juices are a better choice if you do not have the time to juice your own vegetables.

"The choices you make today

Are the consequences you will need

to deal with tomorrow.

Choose wisely, with the future in mind."

- Rita Panahi, L.Ac.

#11

Easy Cleanse to Reset Your Body

Cleansing is an important part of resetting your body to a fresh new start. You don't have to go to a spa, an expensive retreat or buy expensive products to do a cleanse. Cleansing can be simple and very effective even when done on your own. Of course, if you have the time and the means to go for retreats to do a cleanse, they can be a great experience. Oftentimes however, it's difficult and very costly to do so more than 1-2 times in a lifetime. Your body needs rest from heavier foods at least 1-2 x in a year. This cleanse I am about to share with you does just that - gives your body a rest while cleansing excesses, without making your body go into starvation mode.

Ideally, take 7-10 days to do a cleanse, however even doing a short cleanse for 3-5 days will be beneficial. During those days, follow the guideline below:

DON'TS

No meat – which includes chicken, turkey, pork, duck, beef – basically all animal meats.

No fish.

No dairy – which includes milk, cheese, yogurt, ice cream, salad dressings with dairy.

No chips, chocolates, donuts, breads, pasta, muffins, donuts, crackers.

No alcohol, soda, coffee or black tea.

No nuts or nut butters. No jam.

No sugar.

No iced drinks.

No hot spices such as chili pepper, jalapeño, garlic.

No salad dressings (just lemon juice and olive oil)

DO'S

Drink a minimum of 2-3 liters (64-90oz) of room temperature water every day.

Drink hot or warm water first thing in the morning.

All that you eat and drink must be organic.

Take a high-quality probiotic twice a day, once before bedtime and once upon awakening.

Steps for the Cleanse, based on a 10-Day Plan:

Day 1 + 2 eat ONLY long-grain rice, small beans, vegetables and fruits (mung beans are a good choice for beans).

Day 3 + 4 eat ONLY vegetables and fruits (no bananas, no dried fruits, including raisins).

Day 5 + 6 drink only liquids such as vegetable juice, broth from vegetables, fresh juiced fruits (strongly diluted) and drink slow, herbal teas.

Day 7 + 8 eat ONLY vegetables and fruits.

Day 9 + 10 eat ONLY brown rice, small beans, veggies and fruits.

After completing the cleanse, be careful about what you eat. Don't go directly into poor habits, and introduce harder-to-digest foods such as nuts, meat, fish and cheese very gradually and in small amounts. The purpose of the cleanse is to help reset your body and give you extra encouragement to continue eating healthy with improved choices.

Do a cleanse at least 1-2 times per year.

#12

Eat Organic

Buy organic fruits, vegetables, grains, legumes, nuts, seeds whenever possible. Read the labels in the grocery store or market carefully. The same is true for packaged foods, coffee, tea, and salad dressings as well.

The types of pesticides used on conventional produce can be quite harmful. Pesticides, even in small amounts, build up in the body and over time create bigger health problems. Just because a food is packaged, it does not mean that no pesticides were used. Packaged foods can additionally have preservatives added to them that can be harmful to the body. Whatever has to grow, whether it's grains, tea, fruits, vegetables, legumes, or nuts, has pesticides used during its process before harvesting. Many allergic reactions are not due to the food itself but the pesticide that is used on the food. If you find yourself having allergies every time you eat a strawberry for example, try eating organic strawberries and see if you have the same reaction.

If you travel a lot or eat at restaurants frequently, it can be difficult to eat organic. In such circumstances, just make the best choices with what I have shared in this book and when you are home, be sure to do your best to eat extra healthy and cleanse your body with a lot more vegetables or veggie juices. You can't always be perfect, but you can make up for the unhealthy food when you are able to. Any attempt at eating healthier will support you and the more you do it, the greater the benefits.

#13

Wheat. Bread. Choices Make a Difference.

Wheat is given a bad reputation, but you have to remember that wheat is used in many forms, as muffins, donuts, chips, and crackers as well as bread. And there are many types of breads, and the one you choose to eat makes a difference. Not all breads are the same. Eating a healthy form of bread is good. Eating muffins, donuts, chips and crackers or an unhealthy type of bread is not always good. Bread is a form of carbohydrate and carbohydrates are required by your body to produce energy. Having the right amount and the right kind of carbohydrates in your diet is healthy. However, having the wrong kind and too much of it is not.

Bread in truth does not need anything more than flour, water, salt, and yeast. Of course there can be nuts and seeds or various types of grains in there, but the ingredients should be simple. If you read the label, many conventional breads often have a lot more ingredients that are just for preserving the bread or adding more taste to it. Some breads even have added sugar. The simpler the ingredients, the healthier the bread. Keep it simple and keep it organic.

The healthiest form of bread to eat is "sprouted" organic bread or organic whole-wheat bread rather than white bread. When you are buying bread, read the ingredients carefully. And better yet, learn to make your own organic bread!

#14

Dairy

I need to first define what dairy is and what kinds of foods have dairy hidden in them. I have had people think that only milk is considered dairy. However, for those who are unclear, milk, yogurt, cheese, creamers, half and half, sour cream, ice cream, and butter are all considered dairy (if their source is milk, which in most cases it is). And there are many foods that can have dairy hidden in them, for example salad dressings, milk-shakes, chocolate, biscuits, and cookies, to name a few.

It is best to reduce your dairy intake to a minimum and there are two reasons why. Dairy products *often* come from cows or goats that have been injected with hormones to grow faster, in addition to antibiotics. When you consume their milk (in whatever form it comes), whatever the animal was injected with or has consumed will be transferred to you and impact your health. Unfortunately, what the animals are fed is not always the best quality food or merely grass, but oftentimes GMO-based food mixed in.

In addition to this, every food has an innate 'nature', and the nature of dairy is phlegm producing due to its richness. Because of this it has a tendency to clog up the system if eaten or drunk too frequently. Our body has a certain capacity. To eat or drink a little bit of something sometimes may not impact us too much, but to eat large amounts of something or have it frequently may have a noticeable impact on our health and well-being.

Have you noticed sometimes after having dairy that you need to clear your throat more often? Or have you noticed your sinuses get more congested after eating dairy? Or how about coughing more after eating dairy? These are just some of the more directly noticeable symptoms that may occur after dairy consumption. But there are many other conditions that people struggle with, which they are not aware, of the effect dairy is having on them.

I have seen many people's allergies, headaches, menstrual pain, and heavy menstrual bleeding improve after reducing or stopping dairy consumption.

Craving Dairy?

It's easy to make your own milk substitute. Soak 10-15 organic almonds overnight, and throw out that water. Put the almonds with 1-2 pitted dates and a cup of water in a high-speed blender, and you have just made your own almond milk in less than a minute, healthy and without preservatives. You can do the same with cashews or pistachios as well.

Depending on which country you live in, there are many dairy alternatives already available to purchase, from ice cream made from coconut milk, cheese made from cashews, and yogurt made from cashews, to milk from almonds, cashews, coconut, rice or quinoa grains.

Our choices are based on habits and habits can always be changed. The improvement you feel after changing a habit that is not serving you well will give you even more willpower to make more changes and continue on a healthier path.

#15

GMO Food

G MO stands for Genetically Modified Organism. GMOs are organisms whose genetic material have been altered. Corn, soy, canola are some of the most frequently genetically engineered (at least in the United States). If these products on a label do not specifically state that they are organic, it is most likely genetically engineered (GMO). If you are buying any food that has corn, soy or canola in it, make sure it's organic. All 3 of these foods are hidden in many processed foods such as chips, sauces and dressings or even food bars in stores. Corn can be found as corn oil, corn starch, popcorn, tortilla chips and corn tortillas in processed foods. Canola is used very frequently as an oil for cooking. Meanwhile, soy is found in many products as soy oil, lecithin, tofu, miso or soymilk. Edamame beans are soy beans. If you are eating any products that are made from corn, soy, or canola, be sure that they are organic! GMO foods are not natural to the body and as such the body has a difficult time processing them. It is therefore best to avoid GMO food altogether!

"Start your children off on the right track,

To make their health a priority."

- Rita Panahi, L.Ac.

#16

Fruits Alone

Fruits should be eaten alone, at least 30 minutes before other foods and 1-2 hours after other foods. Fruits generally require only 30-45 minutes to be broken down through the digestive process, whereas most other foods require 2-6 hours.

If you eat fruits after your meal as a dessert, especially fruits that are higher in their sugar content, it will cause fermentation.

Though it may seem like a healthy snack, eating apples and nut butters together is also not the best choice in terms of food combining, especially if your digestive system is already somewhat weak. The sugar from the fruit causes fermentation when eaten with another food that has a much higher time requirement for being broken down, leading to bloating, gas and oftentimes constipation. If constipation occurs more frequently for longer periods of time, it means that toxins stay in the body longer, a precursor for many types of conditions based on Chinese Medicine, such as migraines, aching joints, and low back pain, to name a few.

If you want to have nut butters with something, try celery instead.

#17

Meat

Meat is very hard to digest. Most often, animals are given hormones to grow more quickly along with antibiotics, and all this is transferred to you when you eat them. There is a lot of emphasis put on getting enough protein, however, I have found that people are eating much more protein than is necessary. Proteins help with the structure of the body, while carbohydrates help with the energy of the body. It is not necessary to eat meat as a source of protein 3 times a day with every meal on a daily basis. Often just a few times a week is enough for the body. It will also lighten the load on your body's digestion if you include beans, nuts, seeds, quinoa and many vegetables as your sources of protein.

#18

Oils

Oils are used daily in cooking and there are many to choose from, but not all of them are good for your health. Remember, canola oil is often GMO, if not labeled as organic, and many oils that are called 'vegetable' oil are soy, which is also GMO if not labeled organic. Some healthier choices for oils to use for cooking are coconut oil, sesame oil, safflower, and avocado oil. Olive oil is also a great oil to use, however it's best to put it on your food at the end of your cooking. Since oil is something that is used in almost every meal, it is very important to choose the right one and be sure it's organic as well.

#19

It's All About Choices

Educate yourself and be a wise shopper. Know what you are putting into your body and if it is healthy and nourishing for you or just satisfying your taste. Remember that everything that you put into your mouth becomes a part of you. What you eat is what makes you up, your muscles, your energy and how your body functions. As such, you want to be sure that what you are putting into your body will actually enhance your body and health long term, rather than simply give you temporary satisfaction. Your body is resilient and can put up with a lot, but at some point it gives in, which can be the beginning of a lot of suffering. At that point it is sometimes too late and too difficult to turn the wheels back to be healthy.

So the next time you are gravitating towards something that you know is not healthy for you, ask yourself if there is a healthier version and if you are doing your body a service or disservice in the long run. Now you are educated enough to read labels and know the difference between ingredients. Always think of your health in the long run, not only for short term pleasure. Be the master of your body rather than a slave to the cravings and desires.

#20

The Best Time to Eat

In a fast-paced world, it sometimes becomes a habit to skip meals. Or we have the impression that if we skip a meal, it will help us to lose weight. However, based on Chinese Medicine, the body requires the regularity of 3 meals a day minimum in order to not get the signal that it has entered 'starvation' mode. When we skip meals, the body feels that it will not receive a meal and it has to hold onto its resources, and this in turn makes the body hold onto weight. If it's not holding onto weight because we are not eating enough, then it will gradually weaken the digestive organs over time.

It is best to space out your meals, even if they are small, for the morning, noon and early evening. Make your breakfast or lunch the largest meal and keep your dinner as the lightest meal with the aim of eating before 7pm. Eating late disturbs your sleep and doesn't allow your body to go into deep rest while sleeping. The main process of digestion should occur some hours before going to bed, with sleep time being the time for the body to recover and replenish itself, rather than continue working to digest.

"Knowledge is Power.

Now you have the knowledge to choose the

healthier path."

- Rita Panahi, L.Ac.

#21

Body Products

We often think that all the products that we use on our body do not affect us. Yet our skin absorbs what we put on it and the scents that many of the products have, including the chemicals, can be very harmful. This includes products such as hairspray, hair gel, leave in conditioner, soap, perfume, lotion, face mask, serum, deodorant, face cream, makeup and more. The scent may not be from a harmless essential oil, but rather from various chemicals. The price of a product is not what gives it quality or makes it healthy; instead, the ingredients are what make it healthy. Don't always depend on the store to know whether a product is good for your health.

Do your own research and look up the ingredients before making a decision. Usually the simpler the ingredients, the safer it is for you. When you switch to more pure and organic products, your body will get a rest from having to clear the toxicity from the chemicals and ingredients it doesn't know what to do with. Think long term. Illness does not start overnight. It builds gradually over weeks and sometimes years before it shows itself.

Many people who suffer from allergies don't think about the body products that they are using as being a cause. The scents from the products on a regular basis, when they are not from pure essential oils but more toxic chemical sources, can be the cause of many allergic symptoms among other health issues. Choose your products wisely.

#22

Sleep & Rest

Sleep enough hours every night. Sleep is critical for the body and the cells to be replenished. We live in a world where it seems that doing is more important than being and resting. But life is about balance. There are certain hours in the day with light and certain hours with darkness. It is the law of life to have balance. If we are constantly on the go and active with very little rest, we don't allow our body to recover from the day. It's during the time of rest that the cells renew and your body and energy is refreshed. Health comes through resting, recovering and preserving energy, not only through activity and expending energy. Sufficient relaxation and sleep are needed to maintain balance.

Often people think that it's mainly through diet and exercise that weight loss is achieved, however rest is a critical part of weight loss. Learn to know when to stop and slow down. If you have caught a cold, rest. Don't push yourself to go to work or exercise. It's through resting that your body can collect its energy to fight its way back to health.

If you are having difficulty sleeping, certain factors could be the cause, such as coffee, alcohol, sugar, eating late, very hot spicy foods, or taking vitamins in the evening, to name a few. Though some of these may be soothing and relaxing, such as chocolate or alcohol, they can impact the quality of your sleep.

It's best to quiet your mind and senses before going to bed, avoid watching TV close to bedtime, and avoid eating too late. Let the hour before you go to sleep be a time of peace.

#23

Meditate

Meditate daily to quiet your mind. Your mind not only affects your digestion, but everything else in your life. Your mind is the key to feeling peaceful. When you stop everything for 5 minutes a day and even become quiet enough to stop the thoughts in your mind, you can experience very deep relaxation and clarity. It doesn't matter what style of meditation you choose to do. Do what feels comfortable.

As an example, you can just sit on the floor or on a chair or even lay down if that is the most comfortable position for you, and imagine a blue sky, a vast blue sky. Let your mind be the blue sky - vast, clear, peaceful. Allow yourself to breathe gently and naturally as you do this. No need to be hard on yourself if thoughts come or feelings come. Just start again and imagine the blue sky. Your mind is the blue sky.

#24

Exercise & Stretch

Exercise and stretching are like balancing Yin and Yang. Exercise at least 2-3x per week. Your body needs fresh oxygen for all of its functions. Simply walking for 20-30 minutes is good for you to improve circulation and increase oxygen flow into your lungs and body. However, many people only exercise without stretching or with only a little bit of stretching. Exercising tightens the muscles, whether it's cardio, weights, tennis, or whatever it is that you do. Prior to and after exercising, it is very important to stretch out the muscles gently and allow for relaxation and flow. Life is about balance. Over-tightness reduces flow. Relaxation improves flow. It is the flow and moisture within the branches of the tree that make it more flexible to bend. Without flow, the branches become brittle and break. Metaphorically we too become more brittle and more prone to injuries if we don't balance stretching alongside exercising. Stretching not only allows for relaxation of the body, but also more flow in your life and your mind.

It's important to develop the habit early on and continue on throughout your life so that your body remains more flexible. Let stretching, even for just 5 minutes a day, be part of your daily routine. It can be done before you go to bed, at the gym, when you wake up in the morning, or even at work.

#25

Breathe Deeply

Bring oxygen deep into your body with your breath. We have a tendency to breathe very shallow, with the air reaching only to the upper part of our chest. Whether you are at work or at home, remind yourself a few times a day to breathe deeply down into your abdomen. Take in the fresh air and take in life. Your breath is your life. We can go without eating for many days and without drinking for many hours, but we cannot go without breathing for very long at all. Breathing deeply relaxes your body more fully, improves circulation and helps your body to function better.

#26

Stress – the Root of All Disease

Stress can come from many sources, such as work, responsibilities, emotional distress, trauma and more. Stress disrupts the flow of energy within the body. A stressful person is a wound-up person. When you are stressed, everything in your body becomes tight. The solution to this stress is not to drink, smoke, do drugs, or overeat. Instead, the solution is to change your lifestyle to reduce the stress. Often the methods used for reducing stress actually cause more stress to the body long term. Alcohol may relax you in the moment, but long term it will cause strain on your liver and create a new stress as a result of the weakening of the liver's qi or energy. Smoking may relax you at the moment, but long term, it is putting a strain on your lungs and liver and weakening their qi, not to mention building more toxicity in the body. Eating may give you comfort at the moment, but if it's the wrong food, filled with sugar, it will make you feel worse afterwards. So, stress is a cause of many illnesses and the way it's handled is the key to many positive changes towards health.

If you are stressed, don't add more stress to your body, but take a moment to breathe, to go for a walk, to do something healthy for yourself. Get a massage. Sit under a tree. Meditate for 5 minutes. Exercise. Pray. Get acupuncture. Take time off if you are able to. Take care of YOU! You are all that you have. If you fall apart, if your health falls apart, not only will you suffer for a long time, but so will your family, your spouse, your children, your parents and friends. Find out what healthy thing makes you happy and make a point of doing it 1-2 times, if not more, a month. You deserve it.

Think long term when it comes to your health, not short term. The wrong choices today will have long-term repercussions tomorrow.

"Make friends with your body.

Listen to it. Love it. Care for it.

It is your only friend.

But it can turn against you if you don't

take care of it."

- Rita Panahi, L.Ac.

Get your FREE summarized chart of this book

Send an email to:

ownyourhealth@ritapanahi.com

Stay Connected:

Facebook:

https://www.facebook.com/RitaPanahiAuthor/

Instagram: rita_lac

Wishing you the will power and strength to make the right choices, to love your self and take good care of yourself. There is nothing more precious than your health. I know you can do it. Just take it one step at a time and do only one change at a time. Before you know it, you will have turned your health in the right direction.

With love,
Rita Panahi, L.Ac.

About the Author

Rita Panahi, L.Ac., Dipl.O.M., holds a Masters in Chinese Medicine with 3000+ hours of pre and post-Masters training. Over the past decade, she has trained under renowned masters in the ancient teachings of Chinese Medicine rarely found in traditional training programs. She is licensed by the California Acupuncture Board, New York Board and the National Commission of Acupuncture and Oriental Medicine.

She has compiled her vast knowledge and experience to deliver the powerful tips and strategies found within *Own Your Health, Change Your Destiny: Ancient Knowledge Made Simple*.

Also by Rita Panahi, L.Ac.

'Lose Weight Unleash Your Creativity'

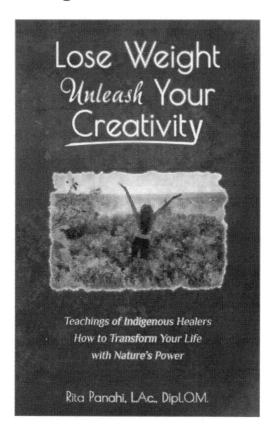

Made in the USA
San Bernardino, CA
08 December 2018